Praise

I like th
offers tha...
understand and SIMPLE to apply. Being reminded
of these four disciplines that
intuitively feel right have really aided me in
maintaining the health I want!

>   *--Mike Keil – CEO, The Resource Agency*

"As a nutritionist I am excited to see this truly
simple, doable approach available to anyone who
will take the time to read this short book. The
health problems related to excess weight in our
country are epidemic at this point, and while not
everyone has the chance to work with a
nutritionist, the vast majority of people could
greatly enhance their health by simply making
these four decisions."

>   *--Elizabeth C.*

"Monte says "if the problem is simple, then the
solution should be simple." I've always tried to
make the problem more complicated than it needed
to be until now. The Simple Math Diet has shown
me the common sense solutions that really work!
This is definitely a plan I can commit to. And as
Monte says, "when I fail, "just start again."

>   *--Abigail Uber*

Much of what is in Monte King's "The Simple Math Diet" I already knew somewhat intuitively, but the affirmation is invaluable. I have lost 10 pounds over the last couple of months by simply applying Monte's first principle of not stuffing myself at meals, and dabbling in principals 2 and 4 of exercise and eating real food. I would have never arrived at his 3rd principal of fasting on my own, and though I find it intimidating, I intend to follow through with it. The thought of losing weight and maintaining a healthy weight without concerning myself with carbs, fats, red meat vs. white meat etc. is quite liberating.

--Lloyd J. Plano, TX

Having played on the pro-circuit of weight loss gimmicks for years, it's refreshing to read something so simple and practical as THE SIMPLE MATH DIET. I'm filled with a sense of hope that maintaining a healthy weight is doable after all.

--Tina Keil, Author of Free to Be Beautiful

"It is refreshing to know that someone has compassion for this problem. Not only does society urge us to eat prepackaged foods that causes us to gain the weight, but then discriminates against us for being overweight. We are all guilty of looking at someone who has excess weight as lazy, or ignorant of nutrition sense, or with just plain disgust. The Simple Math Diet presents a straightforward, simple, and compassionate approach to getting on track with your health."

--Victoria Taylor, Franklin, Tennessee

THE SIMPLE MATH DIET

THE FOUR DECISIONS THAT WILL END THE VICIOUS DIET CYCLE

NOTICE

This book is not intended as a medical manual, but as a reference volume only. The ideas espoused here are intended to help you make good decisions about your health. It is not the intent of this book to be a substitute for any treatment that may be prescribed by a physician. If you suspect that you may have a medical problem you are urged to seek competent medical help.

Copyright ©2012 Monte J. King

ISBN: 978-1481124010

CONTENTS

Foreword

Introduction:
Why Another Weight Loss Book?..................... 1

Personal Diet Gamut... 4
Back to Common Sense................................... 5
The Distrust of Experts................................... 7
Who Are the Bad Guys................................... 8
Simple Versus Easy.. 11

Chapter 1:... 13
The Four Decisions that Will
Change Your Life

Decision #1:
"I Will Never Stuff Myself Again"...................... 14
Decision #2
"I'm Going to Exercise 30 Minutes Daily.......... 17
Decision #3
"I will give my digestive track a
day off every week".. 19
Decision #4
"If It Ain't Food, Don't Eat It!"......................... 25
Simple Math... 30

Chapter 2:
Making the Decision to
Never Stuff Yourself Again............................. 34

Reduced Expense.. 34
Increased Energy.. 35
Improved Digestion.. 36
Weight Loss.. 38
Practical Suggestions..................................... 41

Chapter 3:
Making the Decision to Exercise
30 Minutes Daily.. 43

Weight Loss.. 43
General Better Health.................................... 44
Practical Suggestions..................................... 45

Chapter 4:
Making the Decision to Fast Once a Week....... 49

Reduced Expense.. 49
Increased Energy.. 50
Improved Digestion....................................... 51
Weight Loss.. 52
Practical Suggestions.................................... 53

Chapter 5:
Making the Decision to Only Eat Real Food..... 56

Peace of Mind... 57
Improved Digestion....................................... 59
Weight Loss.. 59
Practical Suggestions.................................... 60

Conclusion... 63

Acknowledgments

I find the task of writing these acknowledgments difficult not because I have received little help, but because the influences over the years on my thinking about a common sense approach to this subject have been a thousand off-hand conversations with everyone from the closest friends to practical strangers.

I am indebted to my good friend (and wonderful author/columnist/poet) Ramon Presson for his input in choosing the title of the book. Thank you to Karen Halbert for making the cover photo shoot such an easy, fun, and quality experience.

To all the people who read my unfinished manuscript and encouraged me to finish the book after many years of dormancy, my gratitude.

Many thanks to Shauna Bryan for getting behind this book and helping form a vision for how many people could be helped by having access to a simple plan like this, and for gracing the cover with her lovely smile. My good friend and colleague, Ken Edwards, has been a rock for me in every way for more than a decade. Finally, thanks to my friend Dr. Bart Huddleston who has encouraged me to stay the course both personally and professionally.

Foreward:

How does one convey in a brief foreward the magnitude of a national problem that affects the lives of millions and perhaps even yourself? And, more importantly, how does one respectfully urge those affected not only to hear but act on the message conveyed in Monte King's brief book? Well, it may be one of the most important efforts I will ever make as a physician, so here it goes....

First and foremost, losing weight, whether 5 pounds or 50 , is simply very hard. And no, it is not fair. It only takes a weekend on a cruise or a Thanksgiving with the family to gain 5 pounds, and it will take a month to lose it! Stress eating over a recent divorce can put on 20, and now you are looking at three months to drop those pounds gained if you are lucky. So what do you do? Sign up for Weight Watchers? Juice fast for 30 days? Dive into everyone's favorites of the cabbage diet or the grapefruit diet? It feels like you genuinely have to put life on hold for a month, two, or maybe even three to even have a chance to lose what you gained. Do not lose hope! Monte King, a highly respected counselor and fitness coach, presents to you in these pages a "simple" and effective way to live and lose weight without putting the joys of life on the shelf. The "simple math diet" uniquely combines simplicity and science, motivation for moderation, and flexibility in your choice of fitness.

Second, you are not your main enemy. Our society has deceived itself into believing processed, convenient foods are a better choice because spending less time eating gives us more time to achieve the "American Dream." Many choose Facebook and Tweeting over walking together or jogging with a friend in the park. We have "super-sized" breakfast, lunch, and dinner without even noticing it anymore. Even fasting, a discipline of all religions and eras of mankind, has been sadly omitted from our culture entirely.

Third and finally, as a physician specializing in Pain Medicine and Rehabilitation, I encounter patients every day with the dilemma of excess weight and pain. For some, it is an elite athlete with an extra 5 pounds to lose due to a hip injury. For others, such as a young mother of 4 crying as she puts her bathing suits in the garage sale, she can barely even see straight much less lose the 30 pounds gained since her first child. For these two individuals as well as yourself, Monte King lays out a passionate case for his "simple math diet." However, I will shed his emotion and speak clearly and plainly. The concepts he presents of eating in moderation, regular exercise, chemical-free foods, and fasting are the building blocks of a lasting weight loss that will enhance the mental, physical, and spiritual elements of your life.

You can finally get excited about losing weight because the process itself, not just the pounds lost, will be life-changing. Ready for a change?

Dr. Barton W. Huddleston, M.D.

To learn more about Dr. Huddleston, please go to **Blueskyhealthservices.com**

Introduction:
Why Another Weight-Loss/Diet Book?

I went to pick up my son from school yesterday. As I sat in the pickup line, the van just ahead of me in the next line over was covered with advertisements for a diet nutrition drink that promised to melt away pounds. Earlier that day I turned on the radio and heard first an ad for a well known weight loss plan. I switched the station--an ad came on for a new pill that would block carbohydrates from being assimilated by your body. You see where this is going. I could go on and on, and so could you, listing the appeals we hear every day to try another weight loss approach. I'm not telling you anything you don't already know. We live in a society inundated with weight loss diets.

It's nothing new--I remember my mother when I was in Jr. High eating little chocolate flavored cubes that were supposed to curb her appetite--but it has accelerated and multiplied into a barrage of fad diets, a multibillion dollar industry, with each latest guru telling us he or she has finally, once and for all, uncovered the secret to fast and permanent weight loss. Finally, you can look and feel exactly the way you want in a few short weeks, or months at the most--and maintain it forever. However, the statistics a few years down the road indicating how many folks succeeded, especially in maintaining their goals (if they ever reached them at all) are rather disheartening.

So why join the parade? The phrase "fad diet" is disparaging, and I used it that way in the paragraph above. Of course, every one of these diets claims not to be a fad diet, but rather the finally-discovered secret that will turn out to be no fad at all-- the sensible and sustainable diet that you will be able to maintain for the rest of your life.

I will, of course, make the same claim. The program I will present to you is indeed effective, sensible, and sustainable for a lifetime, the only one, I'm convinced, that is truly sustainable for most people. I think you will shortly see why, and common sense will tell you, "oh yeah, I really could do *that* for the rest of my life". That last sentence is important, especially the words "common sense". I don't know how many times I've seen people try to convince themselves that their latest diet was doable for the rest of their lives. About fifteen years ago or so, a number of us in the office where I worked were all on a popular low-carb diet. I remember so well when one of my closest friends there said with great earnestness (and, I thought, no small measure of relief), "Monte, I finally found the diet I know I can do the rest of my life". What I remember so well was the feeling inside of me when he said it. I doubted it. Outwardly I was supportive. After all, I was on the diet too and trying to convince myself that the same was true for me. But there were common sense doubts from the beginning that I was trying to ignore. And, alas, neither of us was on the diet six months later, and none of the other six or seven well-intentioned folks in the office faired any better. But, hey, "hope springs eternal in the human heart" right. There's always another diet waiting to be tried.

Personal Diet Gamut

The dictionary defines the word "gamut" as "the complete range of anything". Well, of course, I haven't run the gamut of diets available in the Diet/Nutrition section at the local Barnes and Noble. Who could? But I have, like so many people, my own personal gamut. These have included:

1) A diet espousing mega-calories (for me, 4000 a day) eaten at seven meals a day, to include no simple carbohydrates (not even pasta!), and total fat intake not to exceed ten percent of total calories. Sodium was also strictly limited.

2) A diet severely limiting carbohydrates of any kind

3) A diet severely limiting carbohydrates except for one meal a day, and strictly limiting the time limit of any particular meal (and absolutely no snacks between meals)

4) And of course various diets limiting fat intake, some focused more on certain kinds of fats, others more on total fat intake.

I have also read fairly thoroughly

about a number of other diets, thinking I might just come across that magic one that will be just right for me. And I am aware that I'm a rather mild case when it comes to serial dieting. I don't have a severe weight problem. I'm just one of the gazillions of Americans who always wished I could drop 10 or 20 or 30 pounds, that I liked the way I looked in the mirror when I open the shower curtain in the morning, and that I didn't get so winded just walking up a couple of flights of stairs. I also always felt that I wouldn't mind if my clothes fit a little more comfortably without my pants size increasing every few years. All of those things are now true for me, and can be for anyone. And it doesn't need to be so complicated. I will show you the simplest, most doable approach to looking and feeling exactly the way you want to and your own good common sense will say to you, "Of course, why didn't I think of that?"

Back to Common Sense

Let me return to the theme of common sense. I've heard people quip that "common sense ain't so common any more", and seemingly for good reason. Certainly in the arena of how to eat to achieve and maintain a desirable body composition, common sense has been swallowed up in a labyrinth of complicated, hard to sustain methods. I want to steer us back to simplicity and common sense. The plan I will lay out before you will be so simple, you can walk away from the first explanation of it grasping it fully, and, I believe, knowing in your heart that it is right. Throughout this book, I will be encouraging you to listen to that part of you that just "knows" that something is right.

That's why in this book you will not see a lot of statistics. It seems nearly every one of the divergent methods available presents lots of research and statistics to back up the idea that their plan is the one to go with. And they're all convincing if you are inclined to accept statistical research. But once you're convinced by one expert's apparently thorough and unbiased research, you browse the next book in the diet section and find the same kind of convincing research and statistics proving another plan is the way to go. Spend an afternoon sometime doing this. Eventually your head spins, and you don't know who to believe. How could you? Most of us will never have the time or the energy or expertise to do adequate research to see who's right, assuming such a thing were even possible. But there is a solution. This book will show you that there is someone to trust--no not me--you! If only you can learn to listen to the part of you that already knows what to do.

The Distrust of Experts

We all want experts that we can turn to when we've got problems that need to be addressed. Just yesterday, I chipped a tooth playing with my five-year old in the swimming pool. So today I went to the expert, a dentist. I don't have a regular dentist, so I just asked a good friend, and she recommended a dentist she knew who she thought was both good and honest. I assumed that since he was a licensed professional he must have had adequate training, and sure enough he took care of me. I trust most dentists implicitly. Most of us do, unless we have phobias in that direction. But in the arena of diet/nutrition, many of us are becoming jaded. I suspect that nearly all dentists would have done substantially the same thing that this fine young man did with my chipped tooth today. But if I asked ten "experts" what to do about my extra weight, I'm likely to get ten fairly different answers. I might even get some diametrically opposed answers.

How are we to sort through all the different approaches? Since most of us would not be considered experts in the field of diet and nutrition, how can we possibly be good judges of how to go about eating properly when those who are considered experts offer so many radically different answers?

Who Are the Bad Guys?

The confusion all starts when the experts disagree over who are the bad guys? Are carbohydrates the bad guys? Simple sugars? Fats? Only saturated fats? Simply too many calories? Too few calories? One diet suggests that the bad guys are different for different people depending on your blood type. No wonder we're so confused. We've turned the simple act of eating into rocket science. Let's get back to simplicity. The real problem is quite simple: We eat too much. We eat more calories than we burn, and the body stores the excess as fat, simple as that. You already knew that, didn't you? I don't mean to assert that all these other diets don't have some kind of merit, or don't work, or that eating nothing but ice cream would be okay as long as our total calorie intake was low enough. Of course a balanced diet is important. That's just common sense. But it need not be complicated. As a matter of fact, my personal gamut of diets all "worked" for a time. They worked as long as I could stand to stay on them. But eventually, like the overwhelming majority of most people who have tried these and many other diets, I got worn out by trying to stay on each particular diet and gave up. Sound familiar?

If the problem is simple (we eat more calories than we burn), then the solution should be just as simple. It is possible to define the problem simply, and then go off in a complex, non-common sense direction to solve the simple problem. For example, the mega-calorie diet I was once on defined the problem basically the same way I'm defining it. But then it focused so much on the need to increase metabolism that it went off in the direction of lengthy aerobic daily exercise (at least 45 minutes per day with you heart rate in your "target zone") along with lots of calories and minimal fat intake. Did it work? Yes! But my whole life was consumed with trying to stay on the diet. Cooking, eating 7 meals per day, storing food, drinking supplemental shakes, and exercising until I could no longer sustain the regimen (not to mention the expense!).

Enough. What we need is a simple plan that will be the solution to the simple problem. A plan that is sustainable for a lifetime because it is nothing more (or less!) than listening to our own good common sense that has been swept away in the avalanche of recent diet crazes. This book will give you back what has been obscured in the confusion of trying to listen to the swirl of conflicting experts, and provide you with a simple, sustainable plan for eating and exercising to get you looking and feeling the way you want, and staying that way.

In the next chapter, I will lay out a simple four part plan that will free you forever from looking for the next miracle diet. You will see immediately that if you simply adopt this way of living, it can't help but work for you. But first a word about the difference between simple and easy.

Simple Verses Easy

You may have noticed that I have already used the word "simple" many times in what I've said so far. I have intentionally not used the word "easy" . To be sure, the plan I will present to you will turn out to be easier than most diet plans, especially easier to sustain. But "simple" and "easy" are not always synonyms. Running a four-minute mile is really simple: you simply have to run at a certain pace for 1760 yards.

Simple. But not easy for anyone, and perhaps impossible for the great majority of us even with strenuous training.

All discipline requires some effort. The simple plan I am going to lay out will be quite easy for some, while others will find that it requires a good bit of effort, at least at first. I am convinced that anyone who wants to can quite quickly become so comfortable with the plan that it would be appropriate to say that it is easy. But we don't do ourselves any favors by pretending that a goal worth achieving shouldn't require any effort. To put a little different twist on the illustration above, while it is true that most of us could never run a four-minute mile, most of us could achieve a goal of running, say, an eight minute mile. We could even get to the point where running an eight minute mile would be quite easy. With a little discipline up front, the program I will lay out for you could soon be as easy for you as running an eight minute mile would be for a world-record holding mile runner.

Chapter 1:
The Four Decisions That Will Change Your Life

I told you in the introduction to this book that you would be able to walk away from the first explanation of my common sense weight control program grasping it fully. This chapter will succinctly lay out the simple four part plan to get you eating and exercising in such a sensible way that you will know it is right, and then you can forever forget about spending any more mental energy trying to figure out which diet to follow and save that energy for focusing on just doing what you know is right.

Notice that I refer to a four "part" plan as opposed to a four "step" plan. Many fad diets have "steps", where you may start out doing one thing in the "induction phase" and then something a little different in various other stages, usually ending in a "maintenance" phase which you are supposed to follow the rest of you life. My plan does not consist of steps, but really just four decisions that you can make in the next ten minutes and then sensibly discipline yourself to follow from now on. These four decisions are the "parts" or aspects of the plan. I will simply state them here with a few introductory comments. My goal is to help you reconnect with what you already know intuitively as we take a look at the tremendous benefits of making these four simple decisions.

Decision # 1: "I will never stuff myself again"

Talk about common sense. How many times have you walked out of a restaurant thinking, "Why did I do that to myself? I'm miserable". If it were only once a year at Thanksgiving dinner that we allowed ourselves to consume entirely too much food, it might not be much of a problem. But the reality is, most of us do some form of gorging ourselves on a regular basis, and we're so used to it we hardly even notice. Restaurants pride themselves on giving bigger and bigger portions. And we feel like we're not getting our money's worth if we don't eat it all.

The other day I met a businessman

friend for lunch.

As soon as I sat down he said, "Hey, one of my clients is paying for this lunch, so order anything you want." In the past I would have relished the opportunity to order something I would not normally order, like a filet mignon, and then eaten every succulent bite to take advantage of the opportunity. Instead, I was actually more in the mood for a really good burger. I substituted a loaded baked potato for the french fries, not because I thought it particularly better for me, but because 1) I was more in the mood for a baked potato, and 2) while I might enjoy the fries as much in the restaurant, they wouldn't be as good warmed up later. And, as you will see throughout this book, enjoying your food is an important part of the program. Happily, the burger was one of the best I'd ever had, but easily twice a much as I could comfortably eat. And the baked potato I could hardly eat a third of comfortably, so I took half the burger and most of the baked potato home and had a delicious and fully satisfying dinner.

The thing I want to stress is that I

walked out of the restaurant completely satisfied. I didn't count calories or stress about how much fat content (or carbohydrates, or simple carbohydrates etc., etc.) was in the food. I simply didn't eat more than I was comfortable eating. Simple. Common sense. And the reality is I was actually *more* satisfied than I would have been if I had eaten (or tried to eat) all that was on my plate. I ate my food at a nice leisurely pace, and when I was full, I stopped eating. When I walked out I felt great--full, but not gorged; satisfied physically, and satisfied personally that I had made a wise choice. I knew that I would not spend the afternoon in my office regretting what I had done to myself at lunch. And I knew I was going to enjoy the same delicious meal again that evening--at no cost. As I will go into later, there are many fringe benefits to the program, including a decrease in your food budget, something most of us could really use. This is also satisfying.

I could make the following statement about every decision that I'm going to present here, and probably will. Here's the statement: If you do nothing else that I suggest in this book, do yourself a terrific favor and make this one decision: "I will never stuff myself again". It is one decision you will never regret.

Decision #2: "I'm going to exercise 30 minutes daily"

Again, the common sense of this decision is not going to find a lot of detractors. But at the same time, many people make some kind of decision along these lines often, only to really struggle to stick with it. (Health clubs get an influx of membership sign-ups every year around "New Year's resolution" time). My plan will not take all the struggle away. Discipline is required, but I'm concerned with providing the most doable approach. As I said previously, some will find this rather easy, others will struggle more, at least in the beginning. The reality is that, for whatever reason, some people just enjoy exercise more than others. But one of the problems I see is that often folks make this big decision as a New Year's resolution or at some other time, and unwittingly embark on a program that is going to be nearly impossible for them to sustain over the course of the rest of their lives. In other words, the failure is built in up front because subconsciously they know they couldn't possibly keep doing what they plan on doing forever.

That's why the plan I present is simply to make a firm decision that you will adopt, as a lifestyle, a commitment to exercising 30 minutes a day. This is something nearly everyone can reasonable do for the rest of their lives. After that decision is firmly made, of course you will need some plan to start on right away. But it makes all the difference in the world to know that whatever specific routine you start off with doesn't have to work forever. Most people can't sustain one particular routine indefinitely just out of boredom. On the other hand, sometimes something happens, like a physical injury, that interrupts or even sometimes permanently prevents you from continuing the exercise program you were on. And what happens is that when you unwittingly (this is rarely a conscious thought) put all your "eggs in one basket", then when that particular exercise program becomes impossible or unappealing for whatever reason, you just give up. Much better to make a simple, common sense decision to exercise half an hour as a regular part of your daily life from now on. The decision must be firm, but the method can be, and for most people, must be, flexible.

Decision #3: "I will give my digestive track a day off every week"

Think about it. No fitness trainer tells his clients, "Be sure to work those biceps every single day, we wouldn't want your muscles to have a chance to recuperate, you know". Or how would you feel if you never had a day off from work--at some point your work begins to suffer. Yet most of us go our entire lifetimes practically never giving our digestive systems a day off. I know these are not perfect analogies, but it just makes sense to let your internal organs have some time to rest, to catch up.

I am very aware of the fact that this

is the decision that is going to be the hardest for most people to make.

Everything in our culture militates against it, so much so that when I talk to people about "fasting" a day a week, the typical response is one of disbelief and almost horror at the thought. Disbelief that such a thing would even be possible for them ("I can barely get by skipping a meal--I must have low blood sugar"), and horror at the thought of enduring such a radical ascetic practice. If these are your responses, I understand, I once had the exact same feelings. But do yourself a favor and read on, you might be thankful someday that you did.

First of all, let me address the "doability" of taking one day off per week. That feeling that you have that it would be so hard is simply that--the *feeling* that you can't do something because you haven't done it before. This feeling has no basis in reality. The reality is that fasting a day a week is something that whole people groups have done for thousands of years. These are not special people who just happen to have the ability to fast. The only difference between them and those of us who don't fast is that they have had some compelling motivation to discipline themselves to fast, often a religious motivation. The point is, every person can do it if the motivation is there, and while I'm all for religious motivation, the physical benefits alone, if you will look at them, provide plenty of motivation.

Like I said, I was one who felt like fasting for twenty-four hours would be the height of torture, and that I probably could not do it, but now it's simply a part of my lifestyle, and, believe it or not, something I actually *look forward to* each week. That may sound hard to believe, but once you begin to experience the benefits, the same will be true for you. It's not that I look forward to everything about the fast day--I don't like being hungry--but once I learned to listen to my body, it's as if I can hear my digestive tract pleading "Hey, how about a day off!", and thanking me each week for listening. Again, I don't want to downplay the need for discipline or sound like there is no struggle involved.

I still get hungry on my fast days, and I still have to choose to deny myself, but it can quickly become very manageable for you as it has for me.

The benefits are many. Many people work so hard counting calories and reading labels and denying themselves all kinds of delectable foods, subscribing to all kinds of complicated schemes to reduce calories or fat or carbohydrates only to eventually give up and regain whatever pounds they had lost on their diet of choice, when they could have lost the same amount and established a lifestyle that would keep their results by making one simple decision--to give themselves a day off per week from eating. The first benefits are *physiological*: your stomach, intestines, and colon will thank you; your blood chemistry will benefit from a day off; your kidneys will get flushed (you'll drink plenty of water on your day off!) And of course, you'll lose weight--if you did nothing else but change this one aspect of the way you eat, you would take in one-seventh less calories--that's 14.3%! That's about 100,000 calories a year for the average person.

Common sense will tell you that if you take in 100,000 less calories over the next year, you will very likely be happy with the results.

There are also *psychological* benefits to fasting. For one thing, just doing something that you thought you couldn't do often provides a foundation for doing things in other areas of your life that you thought you couldn't do. For another, many people, including myself, experience a mental clarity and energy that seems to result from having more blood available to the brain rather than allocated to digestive purposes. It should also be noted that, though beyond the scope of this book, many people experience a third area of benefit--a spiritual aspect. In fact, most people who fast on a regular basis do so for spiritual reasons, and it is a discipline that goes back thousands of years in the practice of many spiritual traditions.

If you can get over the initial resistance to the idea of fasting, common sense will tell you that it's just a good idea, with no downside. Once, when I was on a low carbohydrate diet, a registered nurse who specialized in nutrition warned me that the particular diet I was following had been linked to pancreatic cancer, and offered to get me some literature to back it up. I never followed up to get the literature, partly out of laziness, but partly because of what I have said before. I'm sure the research would be compelling, but I'm equally sure that the folks espousing the diet I was on would have their own body of research that would refute such conclusions, and I would once again be left dizzy at trying to figure out which experts to believe. But intuitively, the diet did seem a little strange and extreme, so the comment made me wonder... and fear. What if I was doing something that "worked" in the short run and caused bigger, irreversible problems later? I don't know to this day if that could be true. What I do know is that if someone said to me, "You know, fasting one day a week has been linked to pancreatic cancer", I would smile and say "Oh, have a nice day" and never give it another thought. Or how about, "Never stuffing yourself to the point of misery has been proven to be harmful to your health". Yes, I'm being facetious, because it's hard to imagine anyone even making such statements. Wouldn't it be nice to adopt, for good, an eating and exercise program which would allow you to never again have to wonder for a moment, "Is this really good for me?".

Do yourself an enormous favor: If you do nothing else that I suggest in this book, make this one decision-- "I will give my digestive track one day off per week".

It is a decision that will pay many dividends over the rest of your life.

Decision #4: "If it ain't food, don't eat it!"

"Huh?", you may be saying to yourself at this point, "of course I don't eat it if it's not food. But most Americans have not taken the time to notice, or simply have not been awakened to the fact that we are constantly presented with food that is not food, or certainly not just food. The problem is that the proliferation of low-fat, fat-free and low-carb, etc. diets has caused our grocery shelves to be lined with "food" or, often more appropriately, "food-products" that are filled with chemicals. Much of the food we ingest in this country is filled with stuff produced in a chemist's laboratory rather than grown or raised naturally. Don't be fooled because a product has the word "natural" on the label somewhere. Read the ingredients. A good rule of thumb: if a fourth-grader can read it and recognize it as food, it's probably okay. If you would need to be a chemist to have a clue what half-the ingredients are, put it back on the shelf!

It's amazing how far our culture has drifted from the common sense of this decision. Not a day goes by that I don't hear a friend or acquaintance say something along the lines of "I shouldn't eat this, it's too fattening", or "I guess this is okay to eat, I mean, it's low-fat and all". It's absolutely incredible how conditioned we are to believe that somehow chemicals must be better for us than natural food, because natural foods will make us fat. It's time to face the music--not only does it go against common sense, if we will simply open our eyes we will have to admit it hasn't worked. Dr. Will Clower, in his book "The Fat Fallacy" [1] describes how this reality dawned on him while he was doing his internship in France. He was not studying diet and nutrition, he was studying neurophysiology, but just living in France he couldn't help but notice that the French people didn't worry about eating low-fat, or low-carbohydrate, or low-anything (well, he did notice they weren't big on low-flavor). Coupled with the by-now-well-known fact that the French people experience one-third of the heart-disease rate of Americans and less than one-third the obesity rate, he began to take a hard look at what their country was doing right and what we must be doing wrong. His conclusion: The French diet is big on taste and devoid of fake foods. Their grocery shelves don't have a "low fat" section--they eat slow, they eat smaller portions, they enjoy their meals immensely. And they walk more than we do. Pretty simple.

I heard another commercial driving to my office this morning about that same product that I mentioned earlier--

the one that is suppose to block your body's ability to assimilate carbohydrates. This time, the speaker addressed those who might be listening who were on low-carb diets. He said, (my paraphrase) "Does the thought of eating practically nothing but meat for the rest of your life sound scary to you? Well, now you no longer have to worry about limiting your carbohydrate intake thanks to this amazing new product", and went on to explain how the product blocked carbohydrate digestion. I wanted to jump out of the car. Am I really expected to believe that ingesting a substance that blocks my body from its natural digestive process is *less* scary than eating nearly nothing but meat? The incredible answer to that question is , "Yes, that's exactly what we expect you to believe". And many of us are so conditioned by the message that some natural food, or part of our food, like fats, or, in this case, carbohydrates are the enemy, that we are ready to believe such nonsense, and spend our hard-earned money on ridiculous products. Enough!

Come on, let's reclaim some common

sense in this area. Our bodies are built to run on food. Our digestive systems don't know what to do with chemicals any more than your car engine would know what to do with mayonnaise in its gas tank. For years I have suffered with intestinal problems. I have wondered, "am I lactose intolerant?, should I be a vegetarian?, should I stop eating red meat?, am I missing some enzyme?". Let me say here that I think all of those questions are worth asking, and that things like lactose intolerance are real and I'm not against consulting a physician about these kinds of issues. But I have been amazed at how greatly diminished my digestive tract issues became when I decided to stop trying to put more in my stomach than my digestive system could reasonably handle, and decided I would stop putting stuff in there it didn't recognize as food. Do your body a very common sense favor. Make this simple decision: from now on, "If it ain't food, I don't eat it"!

That's it. Make these four decisions firmly and resolutely, and you will be on your way to a sensible way of managing your physical existence. You will notice that it's not just about weight loss, but about being in shape, about enjoying the wonder of delicious food, about improving your psychological state as well as your physical state. Before long the word "diet" itself will fade from your vocabulary because all you are doing is eating the way your body tells you to once you learn to listen to it correctly. But before we move on, let me show you in simple mathematical terms why making these four decisions can't help but work for you.

Simple Math

The average person eats about two thousand calories a day. Let's just take that number as a good working number and I will show you how simple this is. This is not a quick-fix diet, it's a common sense lifestyle change, so rather than talking about what happens over a few weeks, or even months, let me show you what happens over a typical year.

At two thousand calories a day, the average person takes in 730,000 calories a year. If you make the decisions I have suggested and stick to them, here's what happens: First, about 14.3% of those calories go away immediately because of taking one day a week off from eating. Let's call it 14%, or 102,200 calories. Next, you stop stuffing yourself. I find that the portions that make me satisfied rather than stuffed are barely more than half of what I used to eat, but for the sake of being conservative, let's say your serving sizes decrease by 25%. Of the approximately 630,000 calories left (remember, you've already eliminated 100,000 on your fast day), 25% amounts to another 157,500 calories. Now you add thirty minutes of vigorous exercise to your daily routine, burning about 200 more calories than you would otherwise. Let's say you are only able to average five days a week at this, that's another 52,000 calories. Rounding these numbers down for simplicity's sake, let's see what we've got for a typical year:

Average Intake	730,000
Fast Day	100,000
Serving Size Reduction	-150,000
Burned by Exercise	<u>50,000</u>
Remaining Calories	430,000

You have just eliminated or burned 300,000 calories that your body would have otherwise had to do something with (mostly stored as fat). That's 41% less calories for your body to handle, and all the while you will be enjoying all the delicious, full taste, real foods you love (as opposed to fat-free, low-fat, low-taste, chemical-packed fake foods).

Think about it. Let's say today you and I are sitting on the back porch, both thirty pounds overweight. Now let's say you make the decisions I have suggested and carry them out over the next year, while I just keep doing what most Americans do--routinely overeat, feel guilty, crash diet, fad diet, crash exercise, give up, etc.-- and one year later we're sitting on the back porch again together. Which of us is most likely to be pleased with our physical progress. It's simply not possible that a combination of eliminating and burning

41% of the calories you would normally have ingested will not have a tremendously advantageous effect on your weight and general physical well being. And you will not have spent time and energy fretting over how many calories you were taking in, or what kind of calories. The only label reading you will have done is to make sure what you are buying is actually food. And the physical exercise will produce all kinds of benefits physically and mentally. All you did was make four simple decisions and learn to make them habits--habits, which don't go against good common sense, but which are things your body tells you to do anyway, if you will just listen.

Chapter 2
Making the Decision to Never Stuff Yourself Again

As I mentioned earlier, this decision has a number of fringe benefits. Let's look at a few of them (you might think of a few that I missed).

Reduced Expense

First, there's the reduction of *expense*. Most of us could really use help in that area. I'm sure you have all seen businesses that are focused solely on reducing expenses. I recently saw an editorial column written by a woman who called herself "Mrs. Cheap", instructing people in a weekly column on how to live more frugally. I have heard it said that most Americans are basically two paychecks from living on the street. Clearly most of us could benefit by a reduction in our food bill.

Again, it is so important to look at the long term benefits. If you go to the grocery store today and make a concerted effort to buy less potato chips etc. so you don't eat more, you may only spend $20 less than you normally do. It doesn't seem very motivating, until you do the math and truly let in the fact that when you do that consistently for a year, you have over $1000 extra in your pocket than you would normally have. For most of us, that's not insignificant, enough for a romantic weekend getaway, paying off a debt or some other priority that usually gets put off indefinitely.

But I suspect that the savings involved in this decision, for most people, is most significant when it comes to eating out. Whether it's eating half the food at a restaurant and taking the other half home, or splitting entrees instead of ordering two, the savings in dining out could dwarf the grocery store savings for many individuals and families. When you combine the two, it is likely that over a year's time several thousand dollars could be saved just from making this one simple decision and being consistent with it.

Increased Energy

Another side benefit is the *increased*

energy most of us feel when we eat reasonable portions instead of stuffing ourselves at meals. Most of us are all too familiar with the feeling of needing to take an afternoon nap after eating too much for lunch. I don't know all the science behind this... I suspect that the body is having to allocate so much energy to the digestion process that little is left for other activities. But whatever the case, the fact is that not stuffing yourself doesn't tend to invite the sleep monster to ambush you thirty minutes after your meal, so you are far more likely to have steady energy to focus on the things you want to accomplish.

Improved Digestion

All four of the decisions I'm advocating here contribute to *improved digestion*. Let me stress again that I write as a non-expert. It's simply common sense that when you don't overtax your digestive system by gorging yourself at meals that your digestive tract will benefit. When I was a teenager, there was a popular commercial for Alka-Seltzer where an overweight man sat on the side of his bed in his pajamas with a miserable look on his face repeating to himself "I can't believe I ate the whole thing". The commercial was very effective because everyone of us has had that exact feeling.

When I was 10 years old, I had my first experience with failing to honor this decision. My mother had recently discovered a new recipe for a meal we called "porcupines"--meatballs mixed with rice in a tomato sauce. It quickly became one of my favorite meals, but one night I ate one porcupine too many, to the extent that my stomach muscles separated and something very painfully protruded through my abdomen. I thought I was going to die. Of course, I was fine in a few hours. But while a young digestive system rebounds quickly, a lifetime of over indulging on any kind of regular basis surely takes its toll on a digestive track. One would think that an experience like that might have taught me the lesson to never stuff myself again way back then, but the fact is it took me into my 40's before I made this firm decision. If you're reading this, make it now , whether you are 15 or 75, the time to make this decision is always now, and the benefits begin immediately.

I'll beat this dead horse one more time. Think about it, you get one digestive track, that's it. One stomach, one intestinal track, etc. You have a certain amount of stomach acids to break down the food you take in at any particular meal. Over the course of months and years, when you cut back on the size of your meals and therefore your digestive track isn't in constant overload, it simply has to be of benefit to your ability to digest well.

Weight Loss

Of course the most obvious benefit to many of us will be dropping some unwanted and harmful fat that we carry around. Remember the math at the end of Chapter 1. I'll repeat it here: Most people eat an average of about 2000 calories a day, which means about 730,000 calories per year. I personally find that not stuffing myself usually means eating somewhere between half and three fourths of what would be "stuffing myself". So even taking the conservative number, a 25% reduction in serving sizes over the course of a year cuts out over 150,000 calories from a person's food intake. If you have some unwanted weight and you changed nothing else about the way you eat, common sense will tell you that over a year's time not taking in those 150,000 calories that you normally take in is going to cause you to lose some fat. And all you have to do is make this firm decision and make it a habit.

That last sentence is all important. Remember me talking about the fact that simple and easy are not the same thing? I'm not saying this is easy, especially at first. And especially the part about being consistent. Almost everyone struggles with maintaining good directions in their lives, whether it be better spending habits, eating habits, exercise habits, spiritual practices, etc. But so much hinges on a) how firmly the decision is made, and b) on our willingness to continue to imperfectly struggle toward making a good plan into a habit. This includes the ability to forgive ourselves when we fail and get right back to moving forward.

Some years ago, a friend gave me a book with a curious title, "Always We Begin Again". [2] I was immediately drawn to the title, because it seemed to me to be a graciousness toward ourselves, suggesting that to be human is to be certain to stumble, but that we can always get back up and continue our path. And indeed, that was the basic gist of the book. Interestingly, as I have shared the title of that book with others over the years since, I have experienced two basic, and opposite, responses. Some people respond "That's depressing, you mean I have to start over all the time!", while others have a response similar to what I first felt when I heard it. Not "I *have* to start over", but "I *get* to start over"-- which is good news given that imperfect execution is an inevitable part of being human. Classic glass-half-empty vs. glass-half-full thinking, I guess.

Taking the second attitude is imperative to succeed at any of these decisions. It may sound like a contradiction to some ("If I made the decision firmly enough then I wouldn't have blown it!"). But that is just a refusal to acknowledge your humanness. The best any of us can do is make the decision as firmly as we can, and when we blow it, get up and make it again! And learn from our mistakes (maybe it's best not to order the mega-size meal in the first place if I am trying to eat smaller portions).

Practical Suggestions

Here are some basic thoughts as to how to put this decision into practice.

1. At first, it helps some people to see it in writing every day. Some people put little sticky notes on their bathroom mirror or their computer at work. "Don't stuff yourself"--if it helps you to see it, then by all means write it down where you will see it, make it a desktop background on your computer, whatever it takes!

2. The buddy system is a time tested success formula. Have at least one person who knows you have made this decision (and who you've encouraged to

make it too!), and touch base often.

3. I'll repeat myself here. Do NOT beat yourself up if you blow it. Just be gracious to yourself and recommit to the decision. You'll find this gets easier because now that you have this focus you will be paying more conscious attention to the fact that you're miserable when you stuff yourself, and reaffirming the positive decision to never do that again will come more naturally.

Chapter 3
Making the Decision to Exercise 30 Minutes Daily

Let's take a look at the fringe benefits of making this decision.

Weight loss

It almost feels silly to write this section. There has been so much written about exercise for weight loss that I don't know what I could add. So I'll just restate the obvious: Common sense tells us that if the problem is consuming more calories than our bodies burn, then burning more calories by exercising will be an important part of correcting the problem. The great thing about this decision concerning weight loss is the consistency. The key word is *daily*. Even if the decision results in only 5 days a week, the consistency of regular exercise will have a dramatic impact on your weight, especially if you are significantly overweight. Enough said.

General Better Health

The benefits of daily exercise beyond weight loss are amazing. Again, speaking as a non-expert, but as one who has been involved in regular exercise most of my life, it is clear to me that daily exercise has benefits so far beyond just losing weight that weight loss almost pales in comparison. In fact, there are many who don't need to lose weight who don't exercise, and their bodies and minds are suffering from the lack of regular exercise. Even if we didn't have all the experts telling us about the release of endorphins, increased blood flow, stimulation of all kinds of important glands and brain chemicals, it is obvious to anyone who exercises regularly that you just feel better, have more energy, think more clearly, have a stronger libido. It's not rocket science... a body in motion tends to stay in motion. Oh, wait maybe that is rocket science. Well, anyway, this is another common sense point that we don't need to beat to death. We just need to make a firm decision and make it happen.

Practical Suggestions

1. Pick an exercise routine you *enjoy*. Very few of us are going to sustain an activity we just despise doing. Some people love swimming. I hate it. I know it is a great form of exercise, easy on the joints, etc... people say to me all the time, "it's the perfect form of exercise". I don't care--I hate it, so I'm not going to do it. Fortunately, there are so many ways to exercise, with new ones popping up all the time.

A friend recently told me of a new workout called "Hotbox"--basically kickboxing in a heated room, kinda like hot yoga. Things like that are appealing to me, because I love to sweat as much as possible when I work out, it feels cleansing. But others can't stand the idea. To each his own! Just do *something*, and keep going.

2. This relates to #1. Variety is the spice of life-- for *most* people. There are people who can jog every day for 60 years, if you're one of those, great. But most of us are going to get bored with any routine eventually. So just because

you're really enjoying the routine you're doing now doesn't mean that when you begin to enjoy it less, something must be wrong. Maybe it's just time to explore another form of exercise! I never thought I would enjoy or benefit from yoga, but now it is one of my favorite, and most beneficial, forms of exercise.

One day a friend of mine and I brainstormed about how many different forms of exercise we could do around town, wondering if we could do 30 different exercise forms in 30 days. In less than 10 minutes we easily listed more than 30 forms, from jogging to weight lifting to yoga to kickboxing, pilates, step aerobics, etc. If you're bored with your workouts, look around, there's incredible variety available!

3. Again, repeating myself: When you fall off the exercise wagon, don't waste time beating yourself up. Everyone does it. Just forgive yourself for your humanness (your laziness, your lack of focus, etc.), and forgive the world for being like it is (often it's not your laziness, etc. that derails you, but life circumstances you could not avoid). Just remake the decision to exercise

daily, and start again. Simple. No matter how many times you have to go through that cycle, it's still really that simple. Start again.

4. Similarly, especially as we age, injuries are almost inevitable. It is important to make the decision in such a way as to be flexible. "I'm going to do *some kind* of exercise daily", and make whatever adjustments I may have to make when working through injuries. Many people get married to the particular form of exercise they are doing, and then when an injury forces them to stop that form, they do nothing!

If you are a jogger and have trouble with your achilles, taking some time off jogging doesn't mean you have to sit on the couch until your achilles heals (Ha, get it, Achilles heels/heals). There is almost always some form of exercise that you can do, with appropriate modifications when dealing with an injury.

5. A word about "vigorous" exercise. I have used this word, and I'm afraid it might scare some people because they have a picture of people doing high impact aerobics or olympic weight

lifting, and they know they can't do anything close to either. In reality "vigorous" is defined by your fitness level at any given time. Of course everyone should make sure with a physician that exercise is safe, that is a given. After that, for some people, getting off the couch several times a day is vigorous exercise. I'm not kidding. For others, training for an Ironman triathlon is vigorous. Most of us are somewhere in between, right? So the key is simply (with a doctor's clearance) to choose something that challenges you and do it, 30 minutes a day, and when you improve your fitness you can increase the intensity of your routine. There are times when my fitness takes a step backwards, and I have to adjust what defines "vigorous" accordingly.

Chapter 4
Making the Decision to Fast Once a Week

As I said before, I have no illusion that this is not the hardest sell to people in our culture. People respond with horror at the thought and disbelief that it is even possible. But once we make the paradigm shift and admit that it obviously is possible since many people have been doing it for thousands of years, we can at least begin to entertain the benefits. Let's look at some of them.

Reduced Expense

Just like the decision to not stuff yourself, it's obvious that if you only eat 6 days a week instead of 7, there will be a 14.3% reduction in food costs. This will be difficult to feel at first, but over time, for those who keep fastidious expense records, the difference will be there in black and white. I choose to just simply know it to be true, not being a fastidious record keeper myself.

Increased Energy

You will notice that the fringe benefits of this decision are exactly the same as they are for the decision to never stuff yourself. *Increased energy?* Really? I know it's hard to believe, and it will not feel that way at first.

Remember we're talking about adopting a lifestyle, not experimenting with a fad diet. At first you will feel low energy since your body is not used to being deprived of food for 24 hours. You might even get headaches on your fast day for a while. This is your body throwing off toxins into your bloodstream to be eliminated, something it doesn't normally have the chance to do since it is too busy trying to assimilate what it is constantly being fed.

But over time, as your body becomes less toxic (remember, you're also no longer ingesting chemical/ fake foods), the headaches disappear, the energy is there even on your fast days... you can literally feel you body cleansing itself and enjoying the break from digestion.

Your mind feels sharper (you will likely have many breakthrough ideas on these days as your brain has more energy allocated to it that would normally be needed for digestion). It takes time, but once you are there, you will not want to go back to your old way of never giving your digestive system a day off... the benefits are too important to you now.

Improved Digestion

The ability of your body to digest naturally increases when all of your digestive organs get a chance to recuperate. As novel an idea as this might seem to you if you are considering it for the first time, as soon as you let yourself think about it a little, it's just common sense. You'll have a "why didn't I think of that?" sensation. After a day off, your stomach acids are likely more potent, and certainly less diluted. Another fringe benefit that I'll throw in here is how much better food tastes when you begin eating again the day after your fast day. I call this the Bill Cosby principle. When I was quite young, I remember Cosby talking about how any pleasure is increased the longer you wait for it. He said, "In High School, when I had jock itch I used to wait two weeks to scratch 'cuz I knew it was going to feel sooooooooo good when I finally did!" Hahaha. Well, it was funny when Bill said it. And the principle is true, and a serendipitous fringe benefit of adopting this lifestyle.

Weight Loss

I have referred to this lifestyle as "simple math". I'll just reiterate this here. If you did nothing else I suggest in this little book but make this decision and stick to it, you would reduce your caloric intake by 14.3%, which amounts to a little over 100,000 calories a year for the average person. So along with all the other fringe benefits of improved digestion, reduced food expense, and increased energy, if you changed nothing else about your lifestyle you would inevitably lose some unwanted pounds over time. It really is as simple as that. Not easy, especially at first, but simple and guaranteed to impact your weight in the right direction.

Practical Suggestions

I love to help people who don't think it is possible for them to fast for 24 hours to find out that they can. Here's some suggestions as to how to get there.

1. Ease into it. Start with skipping a meal. If you are someone who has a hard time imagining even skipping a meal... I understand. I've been there. But trust me, you can. Pick a day. Drink lots of water when you feel hungry and just skip one meal, whichever one feels easiest to skip. Over the next couple of weeks, progress to the one that feels hardest to skip. Do this over 3 weeks, then try skipping 2 meals for 3 weeks. After that, you'll be ready to try your first full fast day. Take as much time as you need to get there, just get there!

2. Another way to ease into fasting for a day is to just drink liquids for a whole day. My favorite is juice fasting, which means getting a juicer and juicing your own fresh fruits and vegetables. This has the added benefit of providing live enzymes, vitamins, and

minerals to your diet, something most of us get very little of because almost everything we eat and drink is overcooked or pasteurized.

But even without fresh juicing, just drinking liquids, preferably juices and other natural drinks, gives your digestive track a break from the hard work of breaking down solid foods. Some people like to drink beef or chicken broths. It's a step in the right direction. If you're not ready to tackle a complete fast day yet, try drinking only liquids as an intermediate step, you'll begin to feel the benefits of giving your digestive track a day off.

3. Drink lots of water on your fast day. Most of us don't drink enough water anyway, so here's an opportunity to hydrate to your heart's content. There are several benefits beyond the increased hydration. First, though it will not entirely take away the sensation of hunger, it will partially quell it. This is really helpful especially in the beginning while you get used to fasting.

Drinking lots of water also helps flush your kidneys, and helps flush toxins out of your system. Make sure the water you drink is pure... you don't want to be flushing toxins and adding them at the same time! Again, you can read lots of expert advice about the many benefits of drinking more water, but simple common sense will tell you this is a great idea, and a very practical one when you're not eating!

4. Pick a regular fast day, but be flexible. For most people, it is most helpful to pick a regular day to take your day off of eating. Just pick the day that you are most likely to have the least trouble with. If you go to your mother's every Sunday for dinner, you might want to pick another day. But as with everything else, flexibility is important. If you look on your calendar and realize that there is a special dinner on your fast day, let yourself be flexible and do it the day before or the day after instead of just throwing in the towel on that week's fast. Commitment to consistency is everything when it comes to making these four decisions and implementing them in your life.

Chapter 5
Making the Decision to Only Eat Real Food

When you stop to think about it, we live in a bizarre society in regard to food. Never has there been more information available to us--right at our fingertips-- about nutrition, health, wellness, fitness, etc. And yet the trend toward obesity is staggering. Take a minute and do an internet search of a map of percentage of obesity over the last 40 years in America. It really is hard to take in. And yet in that same time the information available to us about what causes weight gain has multiplied exponentially.

Clearly the problem is not lack of information, or at least not the lack of the availability of the information. But maybe part of the problem is that during that same time, a lot of misinformation was also disseminated by advertisers trying to sell "low fat" diet products. I simply want to point us back again to common sense-- the simple idea that if it's not food, perhaps we shouldn't be eating it. If it didn't have a parent or grow out of the ground, if it was created to taste like food in a chemist's lab, then you should probably put it back on the shelf.

Here's a quick example. Potato chips may not be the greatest nutritional source, but it you look at the ingredients on a bag of plain potato chips, it says something like "potatoes, salt, safflower oil". That's food. Nutritionists will quibble about the harmful effects of frying the oil, and they're probably right, but at least you recognize it as food. But if you buy the flavored chips, or some kind of cheese curls, and you look at the ingredients, you'll see a paragraph of words that (unless you are a chemist) you very likely don't know the meaning of. Maybe food, maybe not. Choose food, something you actually know is food. Simple.

Here are some of the benefits of making this decision.

Peace of Mind

How many times have you watched the news and seen a health report about some additive causing cancer or liver problems, etc. There was the legendary "red dye #2" in the 1950's, and over the years many such products have been eventually linked to health problems. When I was in high school we started putting little Saccharine tablets in our tea instead of sugar, only to hear in a few years that they might increase your chances of cancer. I read articles about additives like aspartame, which seems to be in almost every stick of gum on the counters, and there are concerns. Is it really dangerous? I don't really know. I'm not an expert (did I mention that?). What I do know is that while sugar may not be the best nutritional source, it did grow out of the ground naturally, at least in it's original form. The less processed the better, to be sure, but I'll take sugar over aspartame every day of the week and have peace of mind that I'm not ingesting something that I'm going to find out is fundamentally dangerous tomorrow on the news. Simple. Common sense. Surely we will all sleep better knowing we're not ingesting chemicals that may or may not be harmful to our bodies.

Improved Digestion

I said before that our bodies were meant to digest food. It makes a lot of sense to me that if I put something in my body, especially on a regular basis, that isn't really food, there's a good chance my body is not going to know what to do with it. I'm sure there are all kinds of reasons for troubled digestive systems--I mentioned earlier that I used to have a lot more trouble than I do now. Lactose intolerance is a real thing, and many other issues, but for the great majority of us, making the decision to not eat chemicals and other forms of nonfood is a simple decision that can't help but pay dividends in improving digestion.

Weight Loss

Here's the interesting point concerning this decision. Most of the products that I'm calling "nonfood" were actually developed as attempts to make food less fattening., to provide a way for people to still eat all they want but get less calories and less fat in their foods. But as well meaning as some of these attempts might have been, in the end the common sense of eating only food got ignored. And, again, though I am not an expert, I have seen literature about how it actually backfires and causes more weight gain. One example is a video I watched on YouTube about "Why Diet Sodas Make You Fat". You can watch it if you want some scientific backing for this idea, or you can just apply the common sense thought, "if it's not food, then my body might not know how to digest it, and it might do harm, including possibly contributing to weight gain". The best way to healthy, sustained weight loss is the plan outlined in this book: Eat only food. Don't eat too much. Exercise regularly, And take a day off eating once a week. Simple. Not always easy, but foolproof.

Practical Suggestions

1. Label reading made easy: If a fourth grader could recognize the ingredients as food, it's probably okay. If

you would have to be a chemist/scientist to know what half the words mean, don't buy it. On some diets I've tried, I used to spend significant time scouring labels for caloric content, how many carbs, how much protein, what kind of fats, and on and on. It was exhausting. Now if I look at a label at all (most of the time I don't need to--an avocado is an avocado), I glance at it for about a second and half. That's about how long it takes to apply the advice I just gave. If it's food, and I think I might like the taste, I buy it. If it's not food, I don't buy it no matter how good I think it might taste. Which, by the way, fake foods don't usually taste that good anyway, especially once you get away from eating them for a while.

2. One of the simplest ways to make sure what you're eating is food and food only, is to eat foods with one ingredient. A banana, an apple, a steak, peanut butter (some of it has added ingredients, but you can buy peanut butter, almond butter, etc. that is nothing but roasted nuts. Glance at the label to see). One ingredient not only

equals real food, but usually real healthy food.

3. Baby steps. I've noticed that over the years my diet in regard to not eating fake food gets a little cleaner each year. I think it's because the more you eat real food the more you *want* real food. Some people can make a radical shift and sustain it, but many people will do better with "baby steps". I rarely drink soft drinks at all anymore, but if you drink diet soft drinks, even a shift to regular is a step in the right direction (unless you are diabetic) in my opinion. High fructose corn syrup is probably really not very good for you, but it's closer to food than aspartame. Perhaps after making that shift, once your taste buds no longer crave fake sweeteners, you'll shift from colas to juices--another step in the right direction.

Conclusion

I've kept this book short on purpose. The plan is simple, the ideas are simple. My hope is that you will be freed forever of searching for the miracle diet that is going to finally help you lose the weight you want or achieve the level of health you want. It requires some discipline, especially at first, but one day, if you do it for a while, it will feel like breathing--something you naturally do because it is what you were designed to do.

Think about it one more time. Of course you were designed not to gorge yourself to the point of misery. Of course the human body was meant to move and not be sedentary on a regular basis. Of course you were not meant to ingest toxic chemicals. And of course (this is the hardest to believe given our culture) your digestive track benefits from being given a break on a regular basis.

I hope the very simplicity and common sense of this little book will cause a collective exhale, so that thousands, maybe millions of people will feel relieved of having to evaluate what to do about their physical well being, and just start doing it. The word *start* is so important. The hardest thing to do in many arenas of life is to start. But here's a plan that is so simple to start. Right now. When you go to lunch today, just don't stuff yourself. Boom! You've started. And as I have said repeatedly, when you fail, simply start again.

The math is simple, the ideas are simple, and the execution is simple. And with a little practice, soon, it may even be easy. There are no products you have to run out and buy to get started, no special equipment or supplements, just common sense behaviors that you can decide right now to start practicing.

One thing for sure: If you make these four decisions and work to get better and better at them, you will certainly feel better, look better, and have peace of mind that you are doing the absolute best thing you can do for your body. You will intuitively know that to be true, and no expert or latest fad diet guru will be able to convince you otherwise.

1   Dr. Will Clower, *The Fat Fallacy* (New York, Three Rivers Press, 2003), pp. 40-44.

2   John McQuiston II, Always We Begin Again (Harrisburg, PA, Morehouse Publishing, 1996)

Monte J. King, Th.M., M.A. holds masters degrees in theology and counseling and has been in private practice for over 18 years in Colorado and Tennessee specializing in relational difficulties of all kinds where healthy connectedness has gone awry. His approach honors psychological, spiritual, and physical aspects of a person's life. .

He grew up in Kansas, Oklahoma, and Texas, and his loves include the Dallas Cowboys, Oklahoma Sooners, Jayhawks basketball, acoustic guitar music, (okay an occasional raunchy rock and roll foray) literature, poetry, and physical fitness.

Monte has had a lifelong interest in fitness and nutrition, starting with playing sports in his youth. Like many young athletes, he struggled to gain weight in his early years, but then found after age 40 that the struggle had reversed. After trying a number of different approaches to maintaining an ideal weight, he came to realize that the best and healthiest approach was to follow a very simple, doable, plan, which he has shared in his book, "The Simple Math Diet".

www.theSimpleMathDiet.com

www.MonteKingcounseling.com